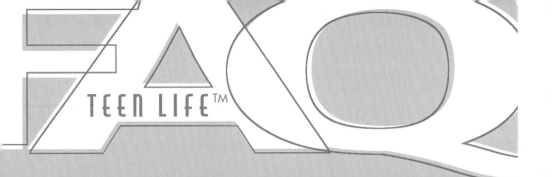

TEEN LIFE™

FREQUENTLY ASKED QUESTIONS ABOUT

Weight Loss

Stephanie Watson

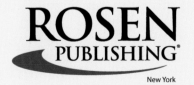

ROSEN
PUBLISHING®

New York

Published in 2013 by The Rosen Publishing Group, Inc.
29 East 21st Street, New York, NY 10010

Library of Congress Cataloging-in-Publication Data

Watson, Stephanie.
Frequently asked questions about weight loss/Stephanie
Watson.—1st ed.
    p. cm.—(FAQ: teen life)
Includes bibliographical references and index.
ISBN 978-1-4488-8328-8 (library binding)
1. Weight loss—Popular works. 2. Weight loss—Miscellanea.
I. Title.
RM222.2.W294 2013
613.2'5—dc23

                                            2012016606

Manufactured in the United States of America

CPSIA Compliance Information: Batch #W13YA: For further information, contact Rosen Publishing, New York, New
York, at 1-800-237-9932.

Contents

1 What Is a Weight-Loss Program? 4

2 Should I Join a Program? 13

3 How Do I Know If a Weight-Loss Program Will Work? 20

4 What Is the Difference Between Dieting and Changing Your Lifestyle? 26

5 Can Dieting Lead to Eating Disorders? 34

6 What Can I Do to Live a Healthy Lifestyle? 46

Glossary 54
For More Information 56
For Further Reading 60
Index 62

WHAT IS A WEIGHT-LOSS PROGRAM?

How often do you think about your weight or wish that you were thinner? How do you feel about yourself when you do think about it?

If you are concerned about your weight, you're not alone. In a 2005 survey published in the *Journal of the American Dietetic Association*, nearly three-quarters of the young women in tenth grade said they had tried to lose weight, and 15 percent said they had begun dieting by age eleven.

Because of our culture's obsession with losing weight, there are countless products and programs that claim they can help you become a thinner and happier person. These weight-loss programs reinforce the idea that the only way to be happy is to be slim—and they say you can't do it without them.

Today, there are thousands of weight-loss centers in the United States. Among the most well known are Weight

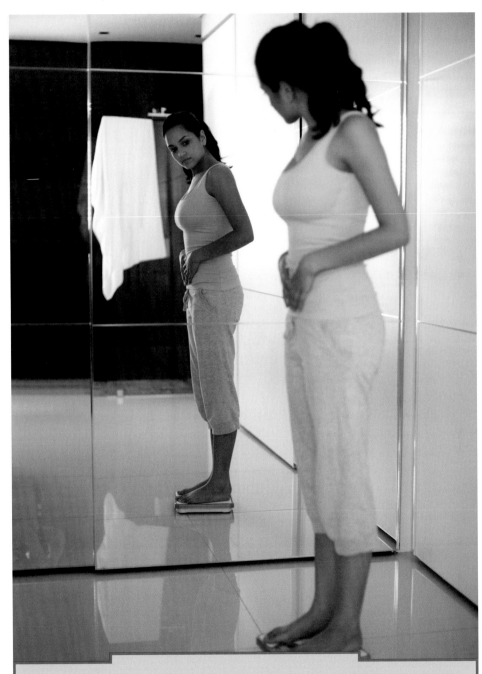

Many girls have issues with their body and weight because of comments from friends, family members, and articles they see online and in magazines. But remember that your weight does not determine your self-worth.

Watchers, Jenny Craig, and NutriSystem. Most likely, you've heard of one or even all three of them. Maybe you've even joined one of them already. Since Weight Watchers started in 1962, millions of people around the world have joined it—some more than once.

Although the details of each program may differ, all weight-loss programs aim to do one thing: to put you on a diet and help you lose weight.

Considering that many people want to lose weight, you may think that there's nothing wrong with helping people do just that. You may ask, "What's wrong with supporting someone who wants to shed a few pounds?" When weight-loss programs tell you that losing weight will make you healthier and happier, it sounds like a great idea. But it's important to listen closely to what these programs offer—and to hear what they're really designed to do.

Types of Weight-Loss Programs

Many different types of weight-loss programs exist. There are countless plans, from do-it-yourself programs to programs that are offered by hospitals and commercial centers.

Clinical Weight-Loss Programs

You can find clinical weight-loss programs at hospitals or through a doctor, nurse, or dietitian. These programs are run by licensed health professionals. They can teach you about nutrition, exercise, and the lifestyle changes you need to make to lose

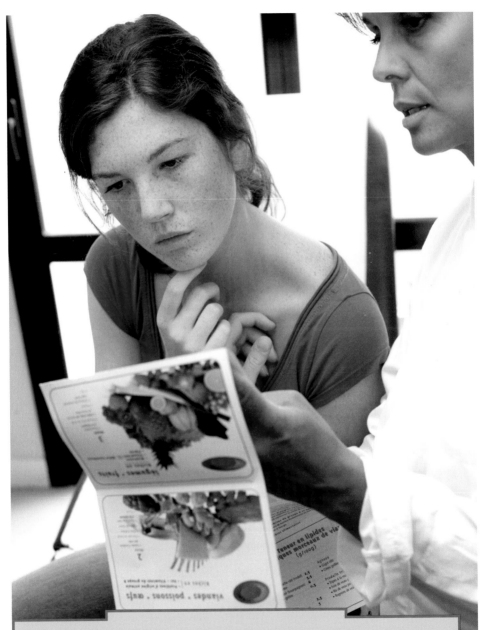

If you are interested in exploring weight-loss options, be sure to consult a doctor or nutritionist who specializes in healthy weight loss. While losing weight quickly is appealing, it can also be dangerous.

weight. For people who are very overweight, clinical programs offer help with very low-calorie diets (less than eight hundred calories per day), prescription weight-loss drugs, and weight-loss surgery.

Commercial Weight-Loss Programs

Weight Watchers, Jenny Craig, NutriSystem, and other commercial weight-loss programs are companies that help you lose weight by various methods. Weight Watchers, which has been a public company since 2001, teaches you how to make better food choices. All of the foods you eat are assigned points. You can eat a certain number of points per day. While on the diet, you meet with a nutritional counselor once a week and get weighed (or chart your weight online). The counselor tracks your progress to make sure you're taking off the weight—and keeping it off.

Jenny Craig (a privately owned company) and NutriSystem (a publicly traded company since 1999) give you calorie- and portion-controlled meals and snacks. You simply substitute their food for what you would normally eat. NutriSystem has different plans for women, men, vegetarians, and diabetics. Jenny Craig gives you access to a consultant, who keeps tabs on your weight and offers you guidance along the way.

In the past, you would go to weight-loss program meetings in your area, but today, many of these programs are also available online. There are also programs that are completely online, such as e-diets. You type in your information, pay a fee, and the Web site creates an eating plan for you and tracks your progress. With online programs, you don't have to be embarrassed about discussing your weight problem in front of other people. You can lose the weight from the privacy of your own home. But you need to have the discipline to follow the diet alone.

Do-It-Yourself Weight-Loss Programs

If you have good self-discipline, you can try one of the many self-directed weight-loss plans on the market. These plans range from books and videos that guide you through a weight-loss program, to prepared meals and snacks you can buy at your local grocery store.

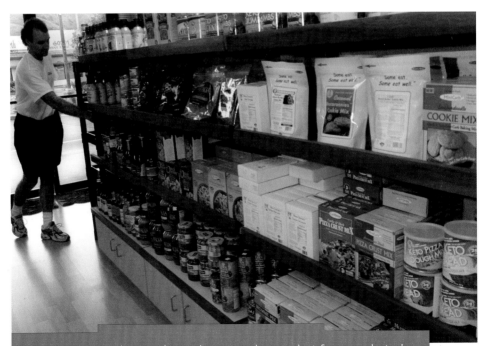

There are many low-carb products on the market for people trying to lose weight. But you must still be sure to check the nutrition information and ingredients before trying them.

Some of the most popular do-it-yourself weight-loss pro-grams today are the low-carbohydrate diets. You probably have heard of the Atkins Diet, the South Beach Diet, and the Zone Diet. The idea behind these diets is that, when your body is low on carbohydrate stores, it starts burning fat for energy. Although these diets can help you shed pounds quickly, some health experts believe they're not the healthiest way to lose weight.

Weight-Loss Support Groups

You can find many weight-loss support groups through commu-nity centers, schools, and churches. The oldest international nonprofit weight-loss support group is Take Off Pounds Sensibly (TOPS). It has been in existence since 1948. TOPS has more than two hundred thousand members in about ten thousand centers around the world. The cost of joining this group in 2012 was between $30 and $36 per year. The idea behind it is to provide members with the support they need to lose weight.

Weight-Loss Camps

Wellspring Weight Loss Camps for children and young adults and other weight-loss camps are places where you can lose weight over the summer months while having fun and meeting new friends. These camps are similar to summer residential camps except that they also offer healthy meals and a lot of high-energy activities to help you get in shape. Some of these camps, such as Wellspring, also offer cognitive-behavioral ther-apy, where teens receive training in goal setting, tracking, problem solving, and stress management to help them in learn-ing healthy eating and lifestyle habits.

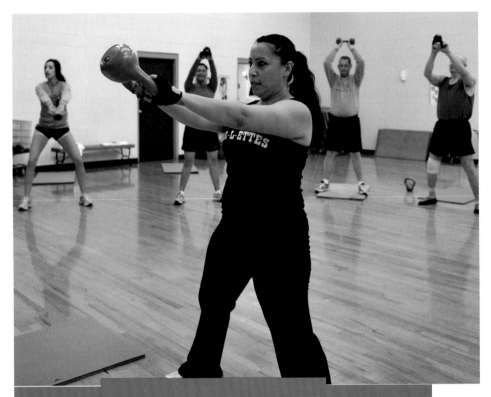

If you are looking to get fit, it's important to find a fitness program that works for you. Many programs focus on aerobic exercise, while many concentrate on building muscle.

Exercise Programs

The YMCA and other community organizations offer fitness and wellness programs for teens. These programs range from aerobics to strength training. They not only give you a great workout, but they also teach you how to exercise safely and effectively when you're on your own.

Myths and Facts

Myth **Weight-loss programs can help you lose weight quickly and keep the weight off.**

Fact ➡ There is no evidence that these programs can help you quickly shed the pounds, or keep it off. The exception is Weight Watchers, which one study did show helped people keep weight off. And losing weight quickly is never a good idea. You want to aim to lose .5 to 2 pounds (227 to 907 grams) per week by making healthy food choices and by exercising.

Myth **A low-carbohydrate diet is the fastest and best way to lose weight.**

Fact ➡ A low-carb diet will probably help you lose weight quickly, but health experts still aren't convinced that it's the safest way to do so. It's much healthier to eat a balanced diet that includes fruits, vegetables, dairy, meats, and whole grains.

Myth **Losing weight is so important that it's worth spending a lot of money on a weight-loss program.**

Fact ➡ Weight loss is about healthy eating and exercise—not spending money. Any weight-loss program that charges you a ridiculously high price is not worth your time. There are many inexpensive options out there, such as community and Internet support groups.

SHOULD I JOIN A PROGRAM?

With so many different kinds of programs available today, it can be tough to choose one that seems perfect for you. Before you make a decision, do your homework. Many programs offer a free consultation if you're interested in joining. They will give you information and help you decide if their program is right for you.

Do I Need It?

Before joining any program, you need to make sure that you really need to lose weight. If you want to shed only a couple of pounds, a weight-loss program probably isn't for you.

Most health professionals will tell you that you need to lose weight if you are overweight and have health problems or if you are obese. You can tell whether you are overweight or obese by finding out your body mass index

(BMI), which is a measure of your weight in proportion to your height. There are special BMI indices for children and teens, which are based on age and gender. To learn more about BMI and how to calculate your BMI, check out the Centers for Disease Control and Prevention Web site. (But keep in mind that the BMI calculation does not factor in muscle and is sometimes considered inaccurate for that reason. See your doctor or nutritionist for the most accurate measurement.)

Talking to Your Doctor

Before you start looking for a weight-loss program, make an appointment to see your doctor. Your doctor will check your weight and general health to see how much, if any, weight you need to lose. Then he or she can refer you to a dietitian, support group, or weight-loss program—whichever is best for you.

What to Look for in a Plan

The ideal weight-loss plan will focus on healthy eating and exercise. Any program that advertises quick and easy weight loss is one to avoid. You should also watch out for any program that pushes diet supplements because these can be very dangerous.

Some things that the National Institutes of Health recommend that you look for in a program include the following:

- A healthy eating plan that includes many different types of food groups
- Slow and gradual weight loss (.5 to 2 pounds [227 to 907 grams] per week)
- Supervision by a counselor or medical professional

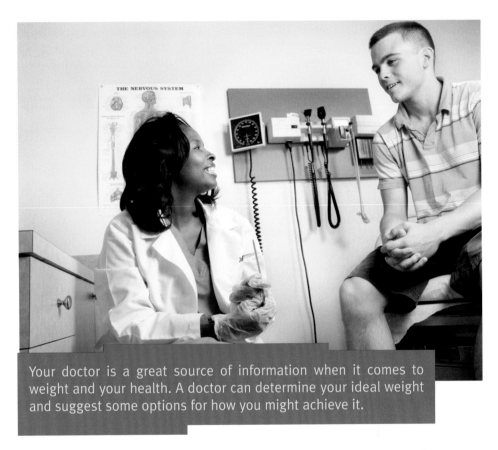

Your doctor is a great source of information when it comes to weight and your health. A doctor can determine your ideal weight and suggest some options for how you might achieve it.

- A plan to help you keep the weight off after you leave the program

A good weight-loss program should be easy to follow and easy to stick with. If you don't think that you'll be able to stay on the diet, consider a different program.

Your Weight-Loss Program Consultation

Usually anyone can join a weight-loss program, whether they are 5 pounds (2.3 kg) overweight or 50 pounds (22.7 kg) overweight. All you need is a desire to lose weight.

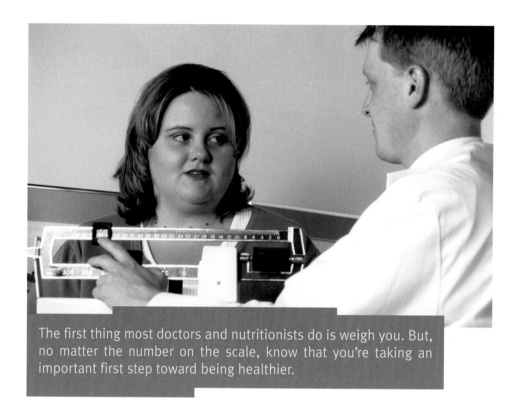

The first thing most doctors and nutritionists do is weigh you. But, no matter the number on the scale, know that you're taking an important first step toward being healthier.

The first time you visit a weight-loss program, you will sit down with a trained counselor to discuss your weight and weight-loss goals. The counselor should have a background in nutrition and exercise, as well as psychology.

The first thing a counselor will do is weigh you, then tell you what your ideal weight should be. Depending on how much weight you want to lose, or how much the counselor recommends that you lose, you'll be given a time frame for your weight-loss goal. This is sometimes called a "personal goal weight." You may not have a say in what kind of program the counselor selects for you. The counselor may pick a plan for you based on your goal. The counselor will tell you that you need to follow the plan exactly if you want to achieve your goal weight.

A counselor will also tell you that the rate of your weight loss is directly connected with how well you follow the program. Many programs claim that you will lose between one and two pounds each week. Counselors suggest that you stay on the program until you learn how to keep the weight off on your own. This could take from six months to a year or longer.

Signing Up

After you and your counselor decide on a plan, it's time to sign up for the program officially. This usually involves paying a membership fee and scheduling counseling sessions. Depending on the program and your age, you may have to bring a parent along with you to sign up. For example, in the United States, you can join a Jenny Craig program when you're thirteen to sixteen years old, as long as you do not have a health condition or take medications and have consent from your parents.

Fees

Membership fees will vary depending on where you live and how long you decide to stay on the weight-loss program. With Weight Watchers, for instance, you pay a registration fee and a weekly fee (about $10 per week if you buy a monthly pass). In addition to membership fees, Jenny Craig charges from about $100 to $140 per week for meals and supplemental snacks. But it sometimes offers special incentive programs, such as "Lose 20

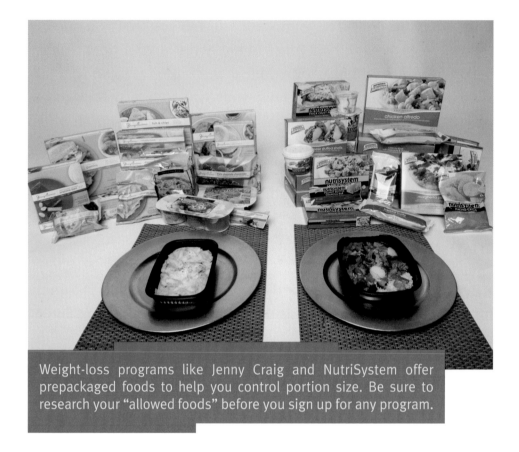

Weight-loss programs like Jenny Craig and NutriSystem offer prepackaged foods to help you control portion size. Be sure to research your "allowed foods" before you sign up for any program.

pounds for $20." NutriSystem has packages that average about $300 per month.

Before you sign up for a program, ask about its refund policy in case you decide to stop in the middle of the program. With Weight Watchers, you pay as you go along, but other programs may require you to prepay and may not refund your money.

Food

The major programs, such as Jenny Craig, Weight Watchers, and NutriSystem, offer their own prepackaged meals. Whether you have to buy the food depends on the program. NutriSystem and Jenny Craig are food-based plans, so you pretty much have to buy their meals. They'll tell you that purchasing their food will give you a better chance of reaching your goal. Your recommended food plan will be very specific and often portion-controlled. This means you can eat only a certain amount of food per meal. Weight Watchers programs give you the option of making your own meals with its recipes or buying its food, which can be found in most grocery stores.

When you join a program that includes food, you are often not supposed to eat out. If you do go out to eat, some programs give you tips for ordering food in a restaurant so that you don't go off the diet. But other programs are extremely rigid about the food and will not allow eating out, especially in the first few weeks of the program. Not being able to eat out can be difficult, especially when you have to watch your friends and family going to restaurants without you.

Counseling Sessions

With most programs, you'll have a counseling session each week to check your progress. The session may be just you and a counselor, or an entire group, depending on the program. You'll be weighed at every session. Your success in reaching your goal is measured by the number on the scale.

Once you've reached your goal weight, the program should start you on a maintenance program to help you keep the weight off. The program may give you informational materials to take home or more counseling sessions. The cost for these counseling sessions varies depending on where you live and what program you join.

HOW DO I KNOW IF A WEIGHT-LOSS PROGRAM WILL WORK?

Weight-loss programs are a business, and, just like any other business, their goal is to make a profit. The staff members of the program are also there to make money. That means they may not always have your best interests in mind when they are designing your plan.

Looking Out for Your Best Interests?

No two weight-loss programs are the same. Although many programs offer a healthy, safe way to lose weight, others may try to pressure you into taking supplements, or engaging in other potentially dangerous activities. That's why it's so important to carefully check out any program you're considering with your doctor. Also

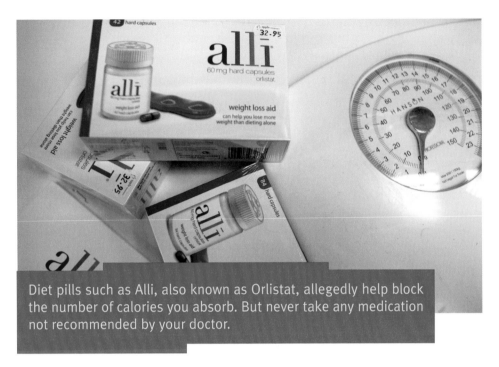

Diet pills such as Alli, also known as Orlistat, allegedly help block the number of calories you absorb. But never take any medication not recommended by your doctor.

watch out for red flags when you join, such as a promise of quick weight loss (more than 2 pounds [0.9 kg] per week).

Diet Pills

In the past, weight-loss centers such as NutriSystem and Jenny Craig made drugs such as fen-phen and Redux available to their clients in addition to diet and exercise programs. Redux is the brand name for dexfenfluramine. Fen-phen is a combination of two drugs: fenfluramine and an amphetamine-like drug called phentermine.

The pills became very easy to obtain. They were also very dangerous, causing heart and lung problems in some users. In September 1997, the U.S. Food and Drug Administration (FDA) decided that the diet drugs could be dangerous and asked the

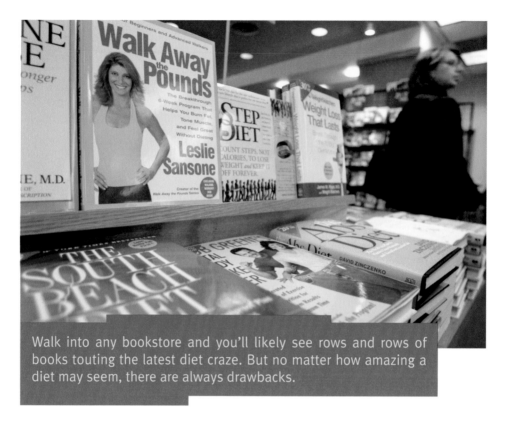

Walk into any bookstore and you'll likely see rows and rows of books touting the latest diet craze. But no matter how amazing a diet may seem, there are always drawbacks.

drug manufacturers to take them off the market. Most of the major weight-loss programs today do not endorse or provide diet pills. If your program advises you to take any weight-loss drug, even an herbal or "all-natural" supplement, don't say yes without first talking to your doctor. Any weight-loss drug you take should be prescribed by your doctor and taken with his or her supervision.

Counselors: Friends or Foes?

Although it may seem that the counselors at weight-loss programs are there to support you, they are often motivated by something else: money. At most programs, the counselors are paid a fee of around $10 to $15 an hour. Most of their income comes from commissions. This means they earn a certain percentage of money depending on how much they sell. The more they sell, the more money they make. The commissions come from sales of the prepackaged food and other materials, such as diet guidebooks, cookbooks, and vitamins.

The counselors who work at these programs usually are not medical doctors. They don't know your medical history. And they often don't ask the right questions. A program counselor should ask you up front whether you've recently visited a doctor about your weight. A counselor should also make sure that you don't have an eating disorder, but not all programs are diligent about doing this.

Weight-Loss Program Realities

Weight-loss programs make big promises. They promise to help you take off all the weight you want, and keep it off. They promise a thinner, more beautiful you. And they promise it will all happen in a short period of time.

Just as with any advertising, you need to be wary of weight-loss program promises. These programs aren't always what they claim to be, and their fees and success rates may not always be what you expect.

Success Rates

All weight-loss programs claim that if you stick with their diets, you will lose weight—and keep it off. If you ask counselors about the success rate of their programs, most will tell you that their program is more successful than any other. But if you ask for proof, you'll find there are few statistics to back up their claims.

There have been only a few scientific studies conducted on weight-loss programs. In 2005, researchers reviewed ten popular weight-loss programs, such as Jenny Craig and Weight Watchers. They found that only Weight Watchers could prove that it actually helped people lose weight and keep it off. Weight Watchers' proof came from a 2004 study it had sponsored. The study found that dieters who had used the program were able to keep off at least half of their weight loss five years later.

One Consumer Reports study that was published in 2003 found that weight-loss programs overall were less successful than losing weight individually. The Consumer Reports survey of more than thirty-two thousand dieters found that most of the people who lost weight and kept it off successfully followed their own program. Only 14 percent of the "superlosers" had ever signed up for a weight-loss program. Most said they lost the weight by exercising.

Your "Ideal" Weight

Many weight-loss programs will tell you that you need to figure out your ideal weight and work toward it. They may use a weight chart to calculate your ideal weight range.

Although a chart can be a useful guide, it can't tell you exactly what you need to do to be healthy. That's why it's important to work with a medical professional, in addition to your weight-loss center counselor, to find your healthiest weight.

Money

It costs a lot of money to join a weight-loss program—as much as a few hundred dollars each month. In addition to the membership fees, there are also prepackaged foods to consider, as well as maintenance programs. A weight-loss program tells you that you need it to teach you how to live a healthy lifestyle. But it will charge you a lot of money to learn. And often after spending all that money, all you may have learned is an unrealistic way to live and eat. According to a report by *Forbes* published by MSNBC.com in September 2006, the top ten most popular diets on the market (Atkins, Jenny Craig, Ornish, NutriSystem, Slim Fast, South Beach, Subway, Sugar Busters!, Weight Watchers, and Zone) had a median diet cost of $85.79 per week, which turned out to be about 58 percent more than the $54.44 that an average American spends on food each week.

Information on living a healthy lifestyle is actually available in many other places for free. You can do your own research on what kinds of foods are good for you. Take a look at the U.S. Department of Agriculture (USDA) MyPlate guide on its Web site. It tells you everything you need to know about the basic food groups and portion sizes. You can also talk to health professionals and read books on nutrition from your local bookstore or library.

WHAT IS THE DIFFERENCE BETWEEN DIETING AND CHANGING YOUR LIFESTYLE?

Food is a huge part of our lives and culture. As the old saying goes, "We don't eat to live, we live to eat." When you try to restrict what you eat, you deprive yourself. Even though you may lose weight in the short term, it's very easy to fall back into your old patterns and put the weight right back on. It's not a diet that you need—it's a lifestyle adjustment.

Eating Realities

You probably don't think about control when it comes to food. When you're hungry, you eat what you want. Sometimes it may be something healthy—other times, you may give in to your craving for some chocolate, potato chips, or a burger. Whatever you decide, you usually

Oftentimes, going on a weight-loss program means giving up some of the foods you enjoy, like burgers and ice cream. But eventually you may be able to add them back and eat them occasionally.

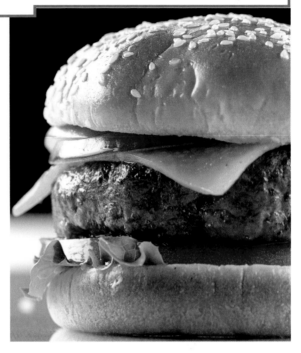

control what you eat or don't eat. But when you join a weight-loss program, that control is taken away from you. The program decides what you eat, when you eat, and how much you eat. When someone else controls the way you eat, it's very natural to rebel. As a result, most people end up breaking the diet they've started.

When you don't lose weight, you often blame yourself and feel like a failure. This can lead to depression and a negative body image. It can also lead to unhealthy attitudes toward food. In the end, you could feel more obsessed with food and weight loss than ever before.

The Trouble with Goal Weights

The most common practice in all weight-loss programs is the "weigh-in." Every time you meet with a counselor or attend a meeting, you get on the scale to check if you've lost weight. And each time the number decreases, you are rewarded. If you are in a group meeting, everyone claps and cheers at the weight you've lost. If you don't lose weight, you may still receive support from the program. However, because so much emphasis is placed on the weight loss, you might feel like a failure or a "bad" person inside.

Because of this emphasis on a goal weight, many people who diet become too focused on a number. Eventually they think of themselves only in terms of their weight. They may forget that there are many qualities that define a person. Qualities like intelligence, a sense of humor, honesty, and generosity may become less important compared to how much a person weighs and what he or she looks like. When all you think about is food and weight, you have less time for the more meaningful things in your life.

The Consequences of Dieting

Your body converts the food you eat into energy. This energy keeps your body going. Your body needs food to survive. When your body does not receive the food it needs to carry on its normal functions, it responds as if it is being attacked. It tries to defend itself by slowing down and conserving energy.

Metabolism Changes

When you skip meals or restrict calories, your body reacts by lowering its metabolism. Metabolism is the rate at which the body burns calories. When your metabolism is lowered, your body stores fat more efficiently. This means as you eat less, your body makes up for the loss by holding on to whatever fat stores it already has. As a result, when you diet for a period of time, and then go off the diet, your metabolism takes a while to pick back up and you usually gain weight again.

Other Body Changes

Although weight-loss programs claim that being overweight can cause health problems, there is strong evidence to show that extreme dieting can also have negative health effects. Lack of food can cause a drop in blood sugar, which can make you feel light-headed and tired. You might also feel nausea and stomach pains.

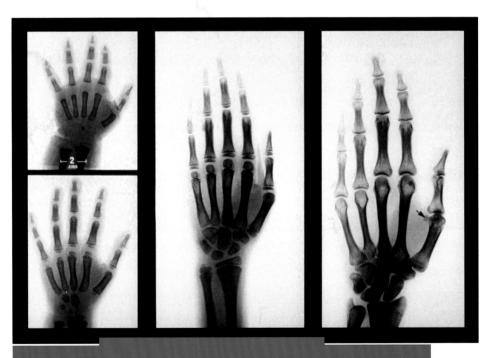

Calcium is a necessary nutrient found in foods like milk and other dairy products. It is necessary for bone development and helps prevent osteoporosis as you get older.

If you deprive your body too much, you may develop serious conditions, such as kidney, heart, and liver problems. Your teenage years are a time when you're still growing and developing. Your body is changing from a child into an adult. It needs energy to make this transformation. If you don't give your body the nutrients and vitamins it needs, it will not develop properly.

For a young woman, a lack of nutrients can cause a delay in her first menstrual period or cause her to stop menstruating. As a result, the lack of estrogen (the hormone that causes menstruation) can lead to a lack of calcium in her body. Having too little calcium could lead to the bone-damaging disease called osteoporosis.

Binge Eating

When you ignore your body's hunger signals and don't eat enough food, your body slows down and begins to function at a level that is below normal. A lack of food can cause you to become irritable and depressed. This depression can trigger the start of dangerous habits, like binge eating.

Binge eating is eating a large amount of food at one sitting. If you binge eat, you often have no control over your eating. A binge can happen when you are on a restrictive diet. You can become obsessed with what you aren't supposed to eat. When you reach the point where you can no longer fight the urge to eat, you start eating uncontrollably, even long after you feel full.

This then sets up an unhealthy cycle of yo-yo dieting. You eat a lot and gain weight, then diet to take it off. Then you begin the process all over again. After a time, your body, as well as your

WHAT IS THE DIFFERENCE BETWEEN DIETING
AND CHANGING YOUR LIFESTYLE?

31

self-esteem, suffers. You may become more desperate in your quest to lose weight. This quest may involve a number of unhealthy behaviors, such as taking diet pills or laxatives, fasting, and exercising compulsively.

Missing Hunger Signals

When you diet too often, you may lose the ability to know when you're really hungry. Your stomach typically tells you when you're hungry. If you've ever been embarrassed by a grumbling stomach, you know what that means. When you deny yourself food, you try to ignore those signals. Soon you can't decide when and if you're really hungry anymore. Instead, you might respond

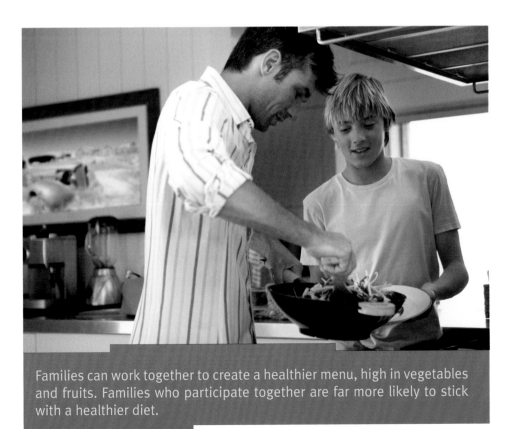

Families can work together to create a healthier menu, high in vegetables and fruits. Families who participate together are far more likely to stick with a healthier diet.

to other, external factors that decide when and how much you eat. For example, you might start to eat because you're stressed out or upset. Although this happens to everyone sometimes, it's unhealthy when it happens all the time.

Fear of Food

Dieting can teach you to fear food. You may start to divide food into categories of "good" and "bad." You may begin to think of yourself negatively if you eat something "bad." Eventually you stop trusting yourself around food. You can no longer tell when you've had enough to eat. You forget that eating is supposed to be fun and pleasurable. You forget that it's OK to eat something because it tastes good. And you forget that food and meals should be positive experiences, not things that make you feel guilty or like a failure.

Ten Great Questions to Ask
When Choosing a Weight-Loss Program

1 Do I need to lose weight?

2 What is my weight-loss goal?

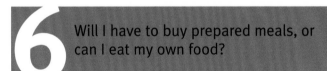

3 What kind of weight-loss program will be best for me?

4 What is the goal of the program(s) I'm considering?

5 Does the program offer personal counseling or group sessions?

6 Will I have to buy prepared meals, or can I eat my own food?

7 How much will the program cost?

8 Does the program include exercise?

9 Who supervises the program?

10 What kind of training does this person have?

CAN DIETING LEAD TO EATING DISORDERS?

Dieting over and over again can sometimes lead people to develop an eating disorder. Studies show that 80 percent of people who have had anorexia nervosa or bulimia nervosa started with a diet. An eating disorder is extremely damaging and dangerous to a person's health. It can cause major physical and psychological problems in a person's life, and it can even result in death.

What Are Eating Disorders?

An eating disorder involves a person's eating habits, psychological issues, and attitudes about weight, food, and body shape. The reasons why a person develops an eating disorder are complex. Someone who has an eating disorder may be experiencing problems with his or her family, job, school, or other relationships.

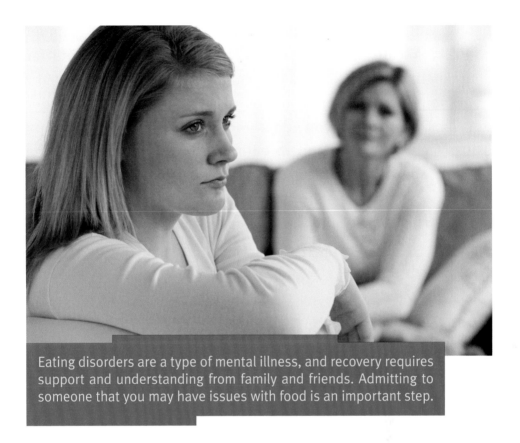

Eating disorders are a type of mental illness, and recovery requires support and understanding from family and friends. Admitting to someone that you may have issues with food is an important step.

The person may have low self-esteem, or he or she may feel out of control in his or her life. Eating disorders are symptoms of these problems. Often, eating disorders start as a way for people to take charge of the one thing they can control—their bodies.

Eating disorders include anorexia nervosa, bulimia nervosa, binge eating, and compulsive exercise. A person can have one or any combination of these four disorders. There are certain characteristics of each disorder, and they all present very dangerous health risks. According to the organization Anorexia Nervosa and Related Eating Disorders, Inc. (ANRED), 20 percent of people with a serious eating disorder who don't get treatment will die. According to one medical expert, the death rate for anorexia that is untreated is even higher, as high as 25 percent.

It's important to understand why and how an eating disorder develops. This way, if you or a friend has an eating disorder, you can get help. The sooner an eating disorder is identified, the sooner it can be treated. ANRED reported that nearly 60 percent of people who have eating disorders and who receive treatment recover from their disorders and can sustain a healthy weight.

Anorexia Nervosa

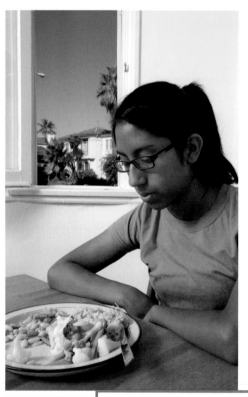

People who have anorexia eat very little or don't eat at all. Because they have an intense fear of getting fat, they literally starve themselves, sometimes to death. They often weigh at least 15 percent below what is considered by doctors to be typical for their height and age. The symptoms of anorexia nervosa include the following:

- Extreme weight loss
- Feeling cold, even in summer

Teens struggling with anorexia find it difficult to even eat a healthy meal with family and friends. They sometimes hide food or just make it look like they ate at least a little.

- Fine hair, called lanugo, all over the body
- Thin, weak bones, a result of the condition called osteoporosis
- Irregular heartbeat
- Lack of fluids, called dehydration
- Depression, irritability
- Unwillingness to maintain body weight

Bulimia Nervosa

People who have bulimia nervosa eat a lot of food at one time (called bingeing) and then get rid of it (called purging) by vomiting, using drugs that cause vomiting, using drugs or enemas to have frequent bowel movements, fasting, or exercising too much. People with bulimia are not always thin—they can be average in body weight or overweight. The symptoms of bulimia nervosa include the following:

- Dry and brittle nails, hair, and skin
- Malnourishment from lack of nutrients
- Cavities and bleeding gums from vomiting
- Dehydration
- Constipation, or difficulty having a bowel movement, from laxatives
- Depression

Binge Eating Disorder

Binge eating is a bit different from the other eating disorders because binge eaters are not trying to lose weight. A person who binge eats may repeatedly eat large amounts of food in a short period of time but not purge. Some binge eaters consume a lot of food in one sitting. Others graze, eating many small portions of food throughout the day and in secret. The symptoms of binge eating disorder include the following:

- Being overweight
- Having constant thoughts of food and eating
- Feeling guilty and depressed about bingeing

Warning Signs

The following is a list of common signs of eating disorders. You don't need to have all the symptoms on this list to have an eating disorder. Do you:

- Constantly think about the size and shape of your body?
- Constantly think about your weight?
- Constantly think about food and about eating?
- Continue to diet after you've lost a lot of weight?
- Not feel good about yourself unless you are thin, but never feel satisfied with how thin you are?
- Feel like you should be exercising even more, no matter how much you are already exercising?
- No longer get your period?
- Limit the amount and types of foods you eat?
- Feel competitive about dieting?
- Force yourself to throw up or abuse diet pills and/or laxatives?

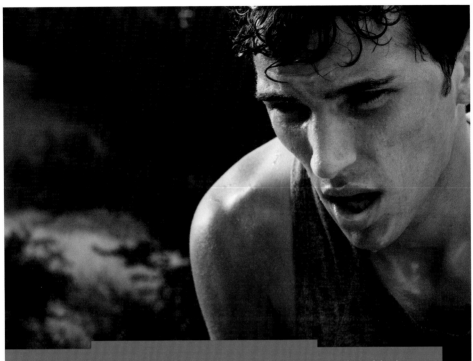

Sufferers of compulsive exercise (also known as anorexia athletica or obligatory exercise) struggle with feelings of guilt and anxiety if they don't work out. Many plan their lives and routines around exercise.

If any of these sound familiar to you, please get help. Talk with someone you trust—a friend, guidance counselor, teacher, or parent. Always remember that you are not alone and you can recover.

What Causes Eating Disorders?

Eating disorders are very complex. There are many factors that together cause a person to develop an eating disorder. Almost everyone overeats or diets from time to time. It's when these behaviors occur again and again that they become a problem.

Who Gets Eating Disorders?

According to the National Eating Disorders Association (NEDA), as many as ten million females and one million males in the United States have an eating disorder such as anorexia nervosa and bulimia nervosa. Although eating disorders mostly affect females, an increasing number of males are developing these conditions. Medical researchers have found that anorexia and bulimia first appear among people who are in their teens or twenties.

The Roots of Eating Disorders

Eating disorders aren't caused by food itself—they're caused by other factors. You probably feel all kinds of pressures from society, your family, and your friends. Television and magazines constantly show images of rail-thin models, and it's easy to want to look that way yourself. Your friends may talk about how they were finally able to squeeze into their favorite size 0 jeans when you're wearing a size 8. And you may have seen one or both of your parents diet to shed a few extra pounds. With pressure to be thin coming at you from all angles, you might feel like you have to start seriously watching what you eat.

Problems in your life—either at school, at home, or with your friends—also can trigger an eating disorder. When you feel like you can't control your life, eating becomes something you can control.

Another major factor for many people with eating disorders is low self-esteem. Not liking who you are on the inside can make you want to change the way you look on the outside.

Getting Help for an Eating Disorder

Doctors treat eating disorders in many different ways. Treatments include therapy, medications, and nutritional counseling. If you are recovering from an eating disorder, you need to find the treatment that works best for you.

Medications

A few types of medications can help you recover from an eating disorder. One is a group of antidepressants called selective serotonin reuptake inhibitors (SSRIs). These include Prozac, Zoloft, and Paxil. SSRIs ease depression, which is common in people who have eating disorders. They can be helpful for people who have bulimia or binge eating disorder. Your doctor needs to be careful when prescribing one of these drugs, though, because they have been linked to suicidal thoughts in some children and teens.

In a large study of drug treatments reported in 2006, four hundred patients with bulimia were prescribed with fluoxetine, a drug that increases levels of serotonin. Those patients who took the drug had fewer instances of binges and purges. However, researchers do not know currently what the long-term effects of fluoxetine will be.

Sometimes doctors prescribe weight-loss drugs such as Xenical for people who have binge eating disorder. These drugs help block some of the fat you eat to stop you from gaining weight. There aren't any drugs that have been shown to be effective in treating anorexia, but behavioral treatments (such as cognitive behavioral therapy) can be very helpful.

Therapy

Therapy is a way to help you come to terms with the feelings that led to your eating disorder. It involves talking to someone—usually a therapist—about problems in your life and feelings you are having. There are many different types of

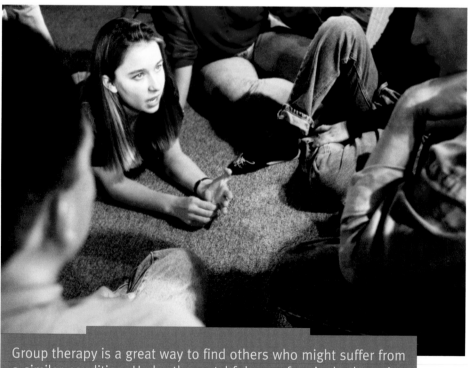

Group therapy is a great way to find others who might suffer from a similar condition. Under the watchful eye of a single therapist, patients can discuss their issues openly with other patients.

therapy: individual therapy, group therapy, and family therapy. Support groups are also a form of therapy. In these groups, you meet with other people who have had similar problems with food. You share your experiences and your ideas that have helped you get better.

Helping a Friend

You may feel uncomfortable talking to a friend who you suspect has an eating disorder. If the situation is an emergency because your friend is really sick or malnourished, you need to get help right away from a teacher, counselor, parent, or medical professional. Otherwise, set up a time to talk to your friend.

Bringing up the subject can be difficult because a person with an eating disorder may be extremely reluctant to let go of the behavior or even admit there's a problem. She or he may become defensive or protective of the dangerous behavior. Be persistent, and get help from a professional if you can't get through to your friend alone. If you know someone with an eating disorder:

- Talk to your friend in a caring, thoughtful way. Try not to express anger or frustration.
- Listen closely to what your friend has to say. Try not to judge him or her.
- Don't fight or argue with your friend. If your friend insists there isn't a problem, say that you hope he or she is right, but that you are still concerned.
- Offer to go with him or her to speak with a counselor or a doctor.

- Don't try to rescue your friend. You cannot save her or force her into treatment. All you can do is say that you are concerned. Your friend must be the one to take the first steps toward getting treatment.

Recovering from an eating disorder can be a long and difficult process that involves many steps. But help is available to those who need and want it. There are many health professionals, organizations, support groups, and resources devoted entirely to eating disorder treatment and prevention. The road is long, but recovery is worth it. In the end, treatment can save your life or the life of a friend.

Improving Your Body Image

These statements, which were developed by Michael Levine, Ph.D., for the National Eating Disorders Association, are meant to promote a positive message. At first, it may be hard to believe or practice some of these messages, but memorize them and repeat them to yourself when you feel depressed. After some time, you may find that they can help you think more positively about yourself and your body. They can even help raise your self-esteem and remind you that you are more than just your weight. Share these statements with your close friends. You can say them to yourself or to each other when you need them most:

- I will remember that being thin will not necessarily make me a happier person.
- I will stop comparing my body with everyone else's.

- I will do things that make me feel good about myself that don't revolve around my body shape and size.
- I will exercise because it's fun, not because it burns calories.
- I will eat nutritious foods because they taste good and are good for my health, not because they'll help me lose weight.
- I will repeat my good qualities to myself every time I feel like putting myself down.
- I will value other people for who they are, not what they look like.

It isn't easy to develop a positive body image. It takes time. But you can eventually learn to feel better about yourself.

WHAT CAN I DO TO LIVE A HEALTHY LIFESTYLE?

Although obsessing about food is unhealthy, it doesn't mean that you don't have to think about what you eat. Weight-loss programs spend a large amount of time talking about what you shouldn't eat. Instead, you should begin focusing on the foods you should eat. What you eat matters—and not just for your weight. Eating nutritious foods will keep you healthy, and it will naturally keep your weight under control. If you change over to a healthier lifestyle, you'll probably find that you don't even need a weight-loss program.

Healthy Eating

It's not easy to eat right all the time. When you're busy, you eat what's convenient and easy. Sometimes your parents aren't around to make sure you're eating balanced meals. Sometimes school lunches aren't very nutritious or

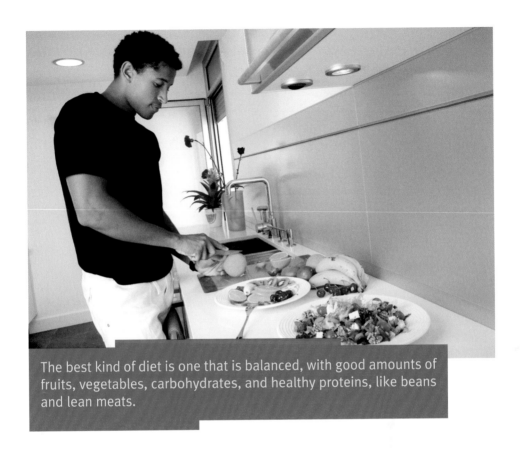

The best kind of diet is one that is balanced, with good amounts of fruits, vegetables, carbohydrates, and healthy proteins, like beans and lean meats.

appealing. But it's important to give your growing body plenty of fruits, vegetables, and protein and to avoid too much sugar, salt, and caffeine.

Nutritional Guidelines

In June 2011, the U.S. Department of Agriculture replaced the MyPyramid guide with the MyPlate guide. This interactive set of guidelines can help you find the right foods and portions to eat based on your age, gender, and how much exercise you get. MyPlate focuses on eating a variety of foods and exercising regularly.

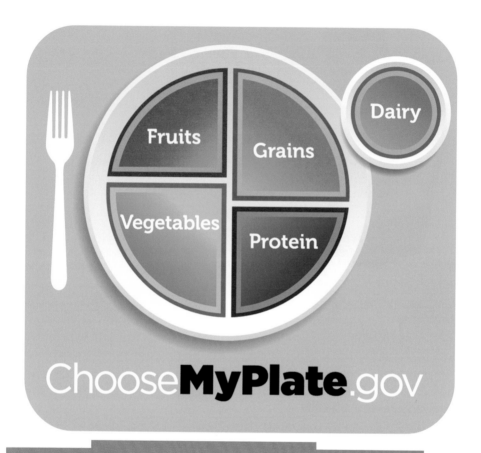

You may have heard in the past of the "Food Pyramid." But many experts argued that it was not the best representation of a healthy diet and replaced it with "My Plate."

Food Groups

You have probably seen or heard about the four basic food groups. This idea was developed in the 1950s by the USDA to try to help people choose the best foods for a healthy diet. It's a simple, smart plan, and its basic guidelines still apply today.

The four basic groups are: milk and dairy products; meat, fish, and poultry; fruits and vegetables; and grains. You need foods from all four groups to be healthy. Let's take a closer look at each group:

- Grains include breads and cereals. The most nutritious grains are whole grains—such as whole wheat, brown rice, and oatmeal. Whole grains give your body plenty of vitamins, minerals, and fiber.
- Fruits and vegetables provide you with fiber, vitamins, and carbohydrates. Fiber helps cleanse your digestive system, and complex carbohydrates give you lots of energy. Many leafy green vegetables contain plenty of calcium as well. According to the MyPlate food plan, you should imagine what you eat during a day as a plate with a cup beside it. Half of the plate would be covered with fruits and vegetables, so they should make up a significant part of your diet.
- Milk and other dairy products—such as yogurt and cheese—are excellent sources of calcium. Calcium helps your bones grow and stay strong, and it keeps teeth healthy. As your body continues to grow, calcium is very important, especially for young women. Fat-free and low-fat milk and milk products are healthier choices than whole milk products.
- Lean meats, fish (especially fish such as salmon and trout, which are rich in omega-3 fatty acids), and poultry are good sources of protein. Protein is important because it helps to take care of your body tissue. Lean red meat is also an

excellent source of iron. Iron helps your body deliver oxygen to body tissues. Strong body tissue gives your body the energy it needs, protects you from disease, and ensures that wounds heal properly. If you are a vegetarian and cut out all meat from your diet, it's important to be sure you're getting enough protein. Nutritionists recommend that vegetarians (and nonvegetarians) eat plenty of beans, soy products, eggs, nuts, and seeds for protein. Sunflower seeds, almonds, and hazelnuts are good sources of vitamin E.

Foods to Avoid

The next time you go to the grocery store, pay attention to the ingredients listed on the foods you buy. The first ingredient listed is the main ingredient. If you see "high-fructose corn syrup" listed first on your fruit juice, it means the drink consists mostly of sugar. It may actually contain very little juice. Many packaged foods, such as TV dinners and deli meats, contain a lot of sodium (salt). Too much salt can drain your body of calcium and can cause high blood pressure and water retention.

Two other ingredients to watch out for are alcohol and caffeine. Not only is alcohol illegal for anyone under twenty-one, it can also drain your body of essential vitamins and nutrients. Caffeine, found in chocolate, coffee, tea, and soda, can dehydrate the body. At first, it may seem as if caffeine is good because it gives you an energy boost, but in the end, it can make you more tired.

Getting Help with Your Diet

It's not easy to follow all those food guidelines, especially when school, work, and social activities can get in the way. You may decide that you need some help in creating a meal plan that works best for you and fits your lifestyle. Your doctor can certainly provide you with information, but you may get the most useful information from a registered dietitian.

A registered dietitian has a college degree and experience in the field of nutrition. He or she has passed a national examination and is registered with the American Dietetic Association (ADA). To find a dietitian in your area, go to the American Dietetic Association's Web site and type in your ZIP code. You can also contact your local health department or search on the Internet for more information about nutrition.

Overall, the most important thing to remember is that eating right is good for your body. Good food makes you feel better, gives you more energy, helps you get a good night's sleep, and keeps everything functioning right in your body. That doesn't mean you can never have any foods with sugar, salt, or caffeine. Most dietitians will tell you that it's a matter of moderation. A balanced diet is a flexible one. It doesn't make anything completely off-limits. But you'll be surprised to find how much better you feel when you eat foods that are filled with vitamins and nutrients!

Exercise

Exercise has so many benefits, in addition to helping you get in shape. Exercise gives you energy and makes you feel more comfortable in your body. It releases endorphins (the body's natural painkillers), which automatically make you feel good. It reduces stress and makes you feel more self-confident. When you make exercise enjoyable, and not something you do just to lose weight, you are more likely to stick with it.

How Much Exercise You Need

The MyPlate guide recommends that children and teens get at least sixty minutes of "moderate to vigorous activity" every day. It should include vigorous-intensity physical activities at least three days a week. Here are some good ways to get that exercise:

- Walking
- Jogging
- Hiking
- Dancing
- Aerobics
- Cycling
- Weight training
- Swimming
- Playing a sport such as basketball, football, tennis, or soccer

Just because you're exercising every day doesn't mean you have to go to extremes. The whole idea is that you should enjoy physical activity. It shouldn't be a chore, and you shouldn't become obsessed with it.

The Best Exercises for You

You can try many different types of activities before you find the one(s) you like. Take a bike ride or go hiking with friends. Go for a fast walk. Ask a friend to come along so you can motivate each other. When there is a choice between taking the stairs or the

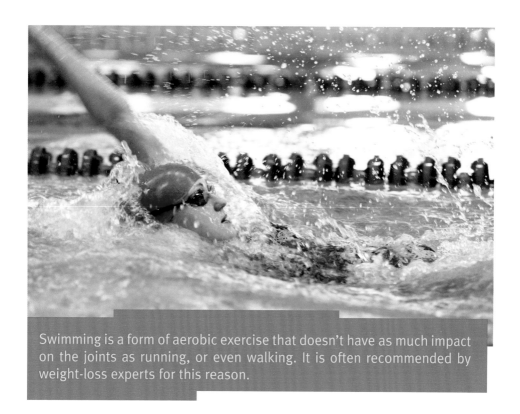

Swimming is a form of aerobic exercise that doesn't have as much impact on the joints as running, or even walking. It is often recommended by weight-loss experts for this reason.

escalator, take the stairs. Instead of driving or being driven somewhere, walk or ride your bike if it's not far.

Join a sport at school or start your own club. If you like to skate inline, start a hockey team. Offer to coach your younger sibling's soccer team. As long as you're moving, you can do anything you want.

anorexia nervosa An eating disorder in which a person eats very little or not at all.

binge eating An eating disorder in which a person eats a very large amount of food in one sitting.

bulimia nervosa An eating disorder in which a person eats a very large amount of food and then purges it from the body by vomiting, extreme dieting, or abusing diet pills or laxatives.

constipation Having difficulty or being unable to have a bowel movement.

dehydration A condition in which the body does not have enough fluids.

endorphin A substance in the brain that can relieve pain and promote a sense of well-being.

fen-phen A combination of the drugs fenfluramine and phentermine; formerly used in some weight-loss programs.

malnourishment A condition in which the body does not have enough nutrients from food.

metabolism The process by which the body uses food to produce energy.

osteoporosis A disease in which the bones become weak and can fracture easily.

portion control A practice that requires a person to eat no more than a certain amount of different types of food.

purge To remove food from the body through self-induced vomiting, over-exercising, or laxative abuse.

Redux The brand name for the drug dexfenfluramine; formerly used by some weight-loss programs.

willpower The ability to control one's own actions; for example, to control how much you eat.

yo-yo dieting Repeatedly going on and off diets.

American Dietetic Association

120 South Riverside Plaza, Suite 2000

Chicago, IL 60606-6995

(800) 877-1600

Web site: http://www.eatright.org

This organization, made up of more than sixty-five thousand members, is the largest group of food and nutrition experts in the country.

Bear Creek Outdoor Centre

45 Barnet Boulevard

Renfrew, ON K7V 2M5

Canada

(888) 453-5099

Web site: http://www.bearcreekoutdoor.com

Bear Creek Outdoor Centre provides different types of events, leadership training programs, and weight loss camps.

Centers for Disease Control and Prevention (CDC)

1600 Clifton Road NE

Atlanta, GA 30333

(800) 311-3435

Web site: http://www.cdc.gov

Information on BMI for children and teens:

Web site: http://www.cdc.gov/nccdphp/dnpa/bmi/index.htm
The CDC is a part of the U.S. Department of Health and
Human Services and provides vital information on public
health and works to prevent and control infectious and chronic
disease and environmental health threats. It also provides
information on nutrition and weight and works to prevent obesity in the United States.

Dieticians of Canada
480 University Avenue, Suite 604
Toronto, ON M5G 1V2
Canada
(416) 596-0857
Web site: http://www.dietitians.ca
This professional society provides information about advancing
your health through food and nutrition.

Federal Trade Commission
600 Pennsylvania Avenue NW
Washington, DC 20580
(877) FTC-HELP (382-4357)
Web site: http://www.ftc.gov
This government agency investigates companies, including
weight-loss centers. It protects consumers from false advertising
and other bad business practices.

International Food Information Council (IFIC)
1100 Connecticut Avenue NW, Suite 430

Washington, DC 20036

(202) 296-6540

Web site: http://www.ific.org

You can find science-based nutritional information created by experts on the IFIC Web site.

Leisure Information Network (LIN)

1 Concorde Gate, Suite 302

Toronto, ON M3C 3N6

Canada

(416) 426-7176

Web site: http://www.lin.ca

LIN is a leading provider, aggregator, and supplier of information and knowledge in recreation, leisure, sport, and healthy living.

National Eating Disorder Information Centre (NEDIC)

ES 7-421, 200 Elizabeth Street

Toronto, ON M5G 2C4

Canada

(416) 340-4156

Web site: http://www.nedic.ca

NEDIC is a nonprofit organization founded in 1985 to provide information and resources on eating disorders and food and weight preoccupation.

National Eating Disorders Association (NEDA)

603 Stewart Street, Suite 803

Seattle, WA 98101

(800) 931-2237

Web site: http://www.edap.org

This nonprofit organization provides information on various eating disorders, including anorexia, bulimia, and binge eating disorder, and helps to find treatment for people with disordered eating.

Web Sites

Due to the changing nature of Internet links, Rosen Publishing has developed an online list of Web sites related to the subject of this book. This site is updated regularly. Please use this link to access the list:

http://www.rosenlinks.com/FAQ/WLoss

Bean, Anita. *Awesome Foods for Active Kids: The ABCs of Eating for Energy and Health*. Alameda, CA: Hunter House, 2006.

Bell, Julia. *Massive*. New York, NY: Simon Pulse, 2005.

D'Elgin, Tershia. *What Should I Eat? A Complete Guide to the New Food Pyramid*. New York, NY: Ballantine Books, 2005.

Gay, Kathlyn. *Body Image and Appearance: The Ultimate Teen Guide*. Lanham, MD: Scarecrow Press, 2009.

Hornbacher, Marya. *Wasted: A Memoir of Anorexia and Bulimia*. New York, NY: Harper Perennial, 2006.

Ingram, Scott. *Want Fries with That? Obesity and the Supersizing of America* (Watts Library). New York, NY: Franklin Watts, 2005.

Lawton, Sandra Augustyn. *Eating Disorders Information for Teens: Health Tips About Anorexia, Bulimia, Binge Eating, and Other Eating Disorders*. Detroit, MI: Omnigraphics, 2005.

Mackler, Carolyn. *The Earth, My Butt, and Other Big Round Things*. Cambridge, MA: Candlewick, 2003.

Orr, Tamra B. *When the Mirror Lies: Anorexia, Bulimia, and Other Eating Disorders*. Danbury, CT: Children's Press, 2007.

Redd, Nancy Amanda. *Body Drama: Real Girls, Real Bodies, Real Issues, Real Answers*. New York, NY: Gotham, 2007.

Schlosser, Eric. *Chew On This: Everything You Don't Want to Know About Fast Food*. Boston, MA: Houghton Mifflin, 2006.

Schroeder, Barbara, and Carrie Wiatt. *The Diet for Teenagers Only*. New York, NY: Regan Books, 2005.

Walsh, Marissa. *Does This Book Make Me Look Fat?: Stories About Loving—and Loathing—Your Body*. New York, NY: Clarion, 2008.

Ward, Elizabeth M. *The Pocket Idiot's Guide to the New Food Pyramids*. New York, NY: Alpha, 2006.

Index

A

aerobics, 11, 52
alcohol, 50
American Dietetic Association, 51
anorexia nervosa, 34, 35, 36–37, 39, 42
Anorexia Nervosa and Related Eating Disorders, Inc. (ANRED), 35, 36
Atkins Diet, 10, 25

B

binge eating, 30–31, 35, 37–38, 41
body image, improving your, 44–45
body mass index (BMI), 13–14
bulimia nervosa, 34, 35, 37, 40, 41

C

caffeine, 50, 51
Centers for Disease Control and Prevention, 14
clinical weight-loss programs, 6, 8
cognitive behavioral therapy, 10, 42
commercial weight-loss programs, 8–9
consultations, 13, 15–17
counseling, 19, 22–23, 24, 27, 33

D

depression, 27, 30, 37, 38, 41, 44
diabetics, 8
dieticians, 6, 14, 51

dieting vs. lifestyle change, 26–32
diet pills, 21–22, 31, 38
do-it-yourself weight-loss programs, 6, 9–10

E

eating disorders, 23, 34–45
e-diets, 8–9
enemas, 37
exercise, 6, 11, 12, 14, 16, 21, 24, 31, 33, 37, 38, 45, 47, 51–53

F

fasting, 31, 37
fen-phen, 21
fluoxetine, 41
food groups, 48–50

H

healthy lifestyle, living a, 46–53
herbal supplements, 22
high-fructose corn syrup, 50

J

Jenny Craig, 6, 8, 17, 18, 19, 21, 24, 25
Journal of the American Dietetic Association, 4

L

laxatives, 31, 37, 38
low-carbohydrate diets, 10, 12

M

maintenance programs, 19, 25
membership fees, 17, 23, 25

menstrual periods, 30, 38
metabolism, 28–29
MyPlate guide, 25, 47, 52
MyPyramid guide, 47

N

National Eating Disorders
    Association (NEDA), 40, 44
National Institutes of Health, 14
NutriSystem, 6, 8, 18, 19, 21, 25

O

Ornish Diet, 25
osteoporosis, 30, 37

P

Paxil, 41
Prozac, 41

R

Redux, 21
refund policies, 18

S

Slim Fast Diet, 25
South Beach Diet, 10, 25
SSRIs, 41
Subway Diet, 25
Sugar Busters! Diet, 25
supplements, 14, 17, 20, 22
support groups, 10, 12, 43, 44

T

Take Off Pounds Sensibly
    (TOPS), 10
therapy, 10, 41, 42–43

U

U.S. Department of Agriculture
    (USDA), 25, 47, 48
U.S. Food and Drug
    Administration (FDA), 21–22

V

vegetarians, 8, 50

W

weigh-ins, 27–28
weight-loss drugs, 8, 21
weight-loss programs
    definition of, 4–11
    joining, 13–19
    knowing if they work, 20–25
    myths and facts, 12
    ten great questions to ask
        when choosing, 33
weight-loss surgery, 8
Weight Watchers, 4, 6, 8, 12, 17,
    18, 19, 24, 25
Wellspring Weight Loss Camps,
    10–11

X

Xenical, 41

Y

YMCA, 11
yo-yo dieting, 30

Z

Zoloft, 41
Zone Diet, 10, 25

About the Author

Stephanie Watson is a writer and editor based in Atlanta, Georgia. She has written or contributed to more than a dozen health and science books, including *Endometriosis*, *Encyclopedia of the Human Body: The Endocrine System*, *The Mechanisms of Genetics: An Anthology of Current Thought,* and *Science and Its Times*. Her work has also been featured on several health and wellness Web sites, including the National Library of Medicine's Medline Plus, BabyCenter.com, and Rosen Publishing's Teen Health and Wellness database, to which she contributed several entries.

Photo Credits

Cover © iStockphoto.com/esolla; p. 5 Yuri Arcurs/Shutterstock .com; p. 7 © Phanie/SuperStock; pp. 9, 11, 22 © AP Images; p. 15 Camille Tokerud/Iconica/Getty Images; p. 16 Carolyn A. McKeone/Photo Researchers, Inc./Getty Images; p. 18 © Jebb Harris/The Orange County Register/Zuma Press; p. 21 Jeff J. Mitchell/Getty Images; p. 27 Josh Resnick/Shutterstock.com; p. 29 Biophoto Associates/Photo Researchers, Inc.; p. 31 Fuse/Getty Images; p. 35 Tetra Images/Getty Images; p. 36 © Bill Aron/PhotoEdit; pp. 39, 47 iStockphoto.com/Thinkstock; p. 42 Zigy Kaluzny/Stone/Getty Images; p. 48 USDA; p. 53 YanLev/ Shutterstock.com.

Designer: Les Kanturek; Editor: Bethany Bryan;
Photo Researcher: Karen Huang